Salmon Recipes Guide for Beginners

Health Benefits of Eating Salmon

By

Bertram Dairmid

Copyright@2023

Table of Contents

CHAPTER 1

Introduction

Salmon, a delectable and nutritious aquatic wonder, has secured its place not only as a culinary delight but also as a powerhouse of health benefits.

1.1 Health Benefits of Eating Salmon

Salmon is a nutritional treasure trove, offering an array of health benefits that make it a standout addition to any diet. Rich in omega-3 fatty acids, particularly eicosapentaenoic acid (EPA) and docosahexaenoic acid (DHA), salmon is renowned for its cardiovascular benefits. These essential fatty acids contribute to heart health by reducing inflammation, lowering blood pressure, and improving cholesterol levels.

Beyond cardiovascular advantages, salmon is a superb source of high-quality protein, essential for muscle development and overall bodily function. Its protein content is not only abundant but also easily digestible, making it an ideal choice for individuals seeking a protein-packed diet.

Salmon doesn't stop there; it's a nutrient powerhouse containing vitamin D, vitamin B12, selenium, and various other essential minerals. Vitamin D is crucial for bone health and immune system function, while vitamin B12 supports nerve function and the production of red blood cells. Selenium, an antioxidant, plays a vital role in protecting cells from damage.

Additionally, the presence of astaxanthin, a potent antioxidant and carotenoid responsible for the fish's pink hue, provides anti-inflammatory and skin-protective benefits. This unique compound sets salmon apart as not just a meal but a holistic approach to well-being.

1.2 Why Salmon is Great for Beginners

Salmon's appeal to beginners in the culinary arena is multi-faceted, making it an excellent starting point for those eager to explore the world of cooking. Firstly, salmon is readily available and accessible in various forms, from fresh fillets to canned options. Its versatility in preparation methods - be it grilling, baking, pan-searing, or poaching - allows beginners to experiment and discover their preferred cooking style.

The forgiving nature of salmon makes it a forgiving canvas for culinary creativity. Its robust flavor pairs well with an assortment of herbs, spices, and sauces, enabling beginners to experiment with different seasonings and sauces to suit their taste preferences. The forgiving nature of salmon means that even culinary novices can achieve a delicious and satisfying result with relative ease.

The quick cooking times associated with salmon make it an ideal choice for those new to the kitchen. Whether preparing a speedy weeknight meal or exploring more intricate recipes, the efficiency of cooking salmon provides beginners with a sense of accomplishment and encourages culinary confidence.

The introduction to the world of cooking through salmon is not just a culinary journey but a health-conscious decision. Its nutritional richness and beginner-friendly attributes make salmon a delightful and rewarding ingredient for those embarking on their culinary adventures.

CHAPTER 2

Getting Started with Salmon

Delving into the world of salmon involves understanding the various types of this flavorful fish. The diversity of salmon species offers a range of flavors, textures, and colors, making it an exciting experience for both culinary enthusiasts and novices.

2.1 Types of Salmon

1. **Atlantic Salmon (*Salmo salar*):**

   - *Description:* Atlantic salmon is one of the most

well-known salmon
varieties. It has a rich,
buttery flavor and a
moderately firm texture.
The color of its flesh
ranges from pink to
orange.

- *Source:* Primarily
  farmed, Atlantic salmon
  is widely available in
  both fresh and frozen
  forms.

2. **Pacific Salmon:**

- *a.* ***Chinook or King
  Salmon*** *(Oncorhynchus
  tshawytscha):*

  - *Description:*
    Known for its high
    fat content,
    Chinook salmon
    boasts a rich, oily

texture and a bold flavor. Its flesh ranges from white to deep red.

- *Source:* Wild-caught in the Pacific Northwest, Alaska, and some parts of Asia.

- b. **Sockeye or Red Salmon** *(Oncorhynchus nerka):*

  - *Description:* Sockeye salmon is prized for its deep red color and robust, distinct flavor. It has a firm texture and is often favored for its appearance on the plate.

- *Source:* Predominantly wild-caught, with Alaskan sockeye being particularly renowned.

- *c. **Coho or Silver Salmon** (Oncorhynchus kisutch):*

  - *Description:* Coho salmon has a milder flavor compared to other species, with orange to red flesh. Its texture is moderately firm.

  - *Source:* Wild-caught in various

Pacific regions, including Alaska.

- *d.* ***Pink or Humpy Salmon*** *(Oncorhynchus gorbuscha):*

    - *Description:* Pink salmon is the smallest and most delicate of the Pacific salmon. It has a lighter color and a more subtle flavor, making it an economical choice.

    - *Source:* Mainly wild-caught, often canned for affordability.

- *e.* ***Chum or Keta Salmon*** *(Oncorhynchus keta):*

- *Description:* Chum salmon has a pale pink to white flesh and a milder flavor. Its texture is softer compared to other salmon varieties.

- *Source:* Wild-caught in various Pacific regions, often used for smoked salmon.

Understanding the nuances of each salmon type empowers cooks to choose the variety that aligns with their preferences and the specific dish they wish to prepare. Whether opting for the richness of Atlantic salmon or the distinct flavors of Pacific varieties, the world of salmon offers a diverse and flavorful palette for culinary exploration.

2.2 Buying Fresh Salmon

Navigating the journey of preparing salmon extends beyond choosing the right type; it involves the careful selection and proper handling of this prized fish.

Selecting fresh salmon is a pivotal step in ensuring a delightful culinary experience. Consider the following tips when purchasing fresh salmon:

1. **Appearance:**

   - Look for firm, moist flesh with a vibrant color. Depending on the species, the color can range from pale white to deep pink or orange.

- Avoid any signs of discoloration, such as dullness or browning, as this may indicate a lack of freshness.

2. **Texture:**

- Gently press the salmon with your finger; it should bounce back, indicating freshness. Any indentation or mushiness could be a sign of aging.

3. **Smell:**

- Fresh salmon should have a clean, ocean-like scent. Avoid fish with a strong, fishy odor, as this suggests deterioration.

4. **Eyes and Gills:**

- Clear eyes and red or pink gills are indicators of a recently caught and fresh salmon. Cloudy eyes or brownish gills may signal age.

5. **Whole Fish vs. Fillets:**

   - When buying a whole fish, the eyes should be clear, and the scales intact. For fillets, check for any discoloration or bruises on the flesh.

6. **Sustainable Sourcing:**

   - Choose salmon labeled as sustainably sourced or certified by relevant organizations. This ensures environmentally responsible practices in harvesting.

7. **Ask Questions:**

  - Don't hesitate to ask the fishmonger about the origin of the salmon, when it was caught, and any other relevant details.

2.3 Storing Salmon Properly

Proper storage is crucial to maintain the freshness and quality of salmon. Follow these guidelines to store salmon effectively:

1. **Refrigeration:**

  - Store fresh salmon in the refrigerator at temperatures below 40°F (4°C).

- Place it on a plate or tray and cover it with plastic wrap or aluminum foil to prevent cross-contamination.

2. **Use Quickly:**

    - Consume fresh salmon within 1-2 days of purchase for optimal flavor and texture.

3. **Freezing:**

    - If not using immediately, freeze salmon in airtight containers or vacuum-sealed bags to prevent freezer burn.

    - Label packages with the date to keep track of freshness.

4. **Thawing:**

- Thaw frozen salmon in the refrigerator or, for a quicker thaw, in a sealed plastic bag submerged in cold water.

5. **Avoid Overcrowding:**

- In the refrigerator or freezer, ensure that salmon is not overcrowded to allow for proper air circulation.

By honing the skill of selecting fresh salmon and implementing proper storage techniques, enthusiasts can embark on their culinary journey with the confidence that they are working with the finest and freshest ingredients.

CHAPTER 3

Basic Cooking Techniques

Salmon's versatility in the kitchen shines through various cooking methods, each imparting its unique flavor profile and texture.

3.1 Grilling Salmon

Grilling is a popular method that imparts a smoky, charred flavor to salmon while maintaining its natural juiciness. Here's a step-by-step guide to grilling salmon:

Ingredients:

- Fresh salmon fillets or steaks

- Olive oil

- Salt and pepper

- Lemon wedges (for serving)

Instructions:

1. **Preheat the Grill:**

   - Preheat your grill to medium-high heat. Make sure the grates are clean and well-oiled to prevent sticking.

2. **Prepare the Salmon:**

   - Pat the salmon dry with paper towels. Brush both sides with olive oil, and season with salt and pepper.

3. **Grilling:**

- Place the salmon skin-side down on the preheated grill. Close the lid and cook for about 4-5 minutes.

4. **Flipping:**

   - Carefully flip the salmon using a spatula. Grill for an additional 4-5 minutes or until the salmon is opaque and easily flakes with a fork.

5. **Serve:**

   - Remove from the grill and let it rest for a few minutes before serving. Squeeze fresh lemon over the grilled salmon for a burst of citrusy flavor.

- Use a fish basket or aluminum foil to prevent the salmon from sticking to the grill grates.

- Experiment with marinades or rubs to enhance the flavor.

3.2 Baking Salmon

Baking is a convenient and foolproof method for cooking salmon, resulting in a moist and tender texture. Here's a simple guide to baking salmon:

Ingredients:

- Fresh salmon fillets or a whole side of salmon

- Olive oil

- Salt and pepper

- Lemon slices

- Fresh herbs (such as dill, parsley, or thyme)

Instructions:

1. **Preheat the Oven:**

   - Preheat your oven to 375°F (190°C).

2. **Prepare the Salmon:**

   - Place the salmon on a baking sheet lined with parchment paper or aluminum foil. Brush the salmon with olive oil and season with salt and pepper.

3. **Flavor Infusion:**

   - Add fresh lemon slices on top of the salmon, and sprinkle with fresh herbs for added flavor.

4. **Baking:**

- Bake in the preheated
  oven for 12-15 minutes,
  or until the salmon flakes
  easily with a fork.
  Cooking times may vary
  based on the thickness of
  the fillets.

5. **Serve:**

- Carefully transfer the
  salmon to a serving
  platter. Garnish with
  additional herbs and
  lemon wedges.

Tips:

- Consider marinating the salmon
  beforehand for added flavor.

- To check for doneness, use a
  fork to gently pull apart the
  flesh; it should easily flake.

By mastering these basic cooking techniques, enthusiasts can confidently prepare delicious and succulent salmon dishes, whether opting for the bold flavors of grilled salmon or the oven-baked perfection that highlights the fish's natural taste.

3.3 Pan-Seared Salmon

Continuing our exploration of basic cooking techniques for salmon, let's delve into the art of pan-searing and poaching. These methods offer different textures and flavors, showcasing the versatility of this delectable fish.

Pan-searing salmon creates a crispy, flavorful crust while maintaining a tender interior. This technique is quick and ideal for busy weeknight meals. Here's a step-by-step guide:

Ingredients:

- Fresh salmon fillets

- Olive oil

- Salt and pepper

- Optional: Fresh herbs (such as thyme or rosemary)

Instructions:

1. **Preparation:**

   - Pat the salmon fillets dry with paper towels. Season both sides with salt and pepper. Optionally, sprinkle fresh herbs on the fillets for added flavor.

2. **Preheat the Pan:**

   - Heat a non-stick skillet or cast-iron pan over

medium-high heat. Add a thin layer of olive oil and let it heat until shimmering.

3. **Searing:**

- Place the salmon fillets in the pan, skin-side down. Sear for 3-4 minutes until the skin becomes crispy and golden.

4. **Flip and Finish:**

- Carefully flip the fillets using a spatula. Cook for an additional 3-4 minutes, or until the salmon is opaque and flakes easily.

5. **Serve:**

- Remove from the pan and let the salmon rest for a minute. Serve with your favorite side dishes.

Tips:

- For extra flavor, add a squeeze of lemon or a drizzle of balsamic glaze after cooking.

- Experiment with different herb and spice rubs for a personalized touch.

3.4 Poaching Salmon

Poaching salmon involves gently simmering the fish in a flavorful liquid, resulting in a delicate and moist texture. This method is excellent for retaining the natural flavors of the salmon. Here's how to poach salmon:

Ingredients:

- Fresh salmon fillets

- Poaching liquid (water, broth, wine)

- Aromatics (such as sliced onions, lemon, and fresh herbs)

- Salt and pepper

Instructions:

1. **Prepare the Poaching Liquid:**

    - In a wide, shallow pan, add enough liquid (water, broth, or a combination) to cover the salmon fillets. Season the liquid with salt, pepper, and aromatics.

2. **Heat the Liquid:**

- Bring the poaching liquid
  to a gentle simmer over
  medium heat. Ensure it's
  hot but not boiling.

3. **Poaching:**

   - Carefully add the salmon
     fillets to the simmering
     liquid. Poach for 4-6
     minutes, depending on
     the thickness of the
     fillets, until the salmon is
     opaque and flakes easily.

4. **Serve:**

   - Using a slotted spatula,
     remove the poached
     salmon from the liquid.
     Serve on a plate, and if
     desired, drizzle with a
     simple sauce or
     additional herbs.

Tips:

- Customize the poaching liquid with your favorite herbs, spices, and citrus flavors.

- Use a flavorful broth or wine for added depth.

Mastering pan-searing and poaching techniques expands your repertoire, allowing you to enjoy salmon in different ways. Whether opting for the crispiness of pan-seared fillets or the delicate tenderness achieved through poaching, these methods showcase the culinary versatility of this prized fish.

3.5 Steaming Salmon

Steaming is a gentle and health-conscious method for preparing salmon that preserves its natural flavors and nutrients.

Steaming salmon is a technique that yields a light and flaky texture while maintaining the fish's inherent taste. Here's how to steam salmon:

Ingredients:

- Fresh salmon fillets

- Lemon slices

- Fresh herbs (such as dill or parsley)

- Salt and pepper

Instructions:

1. **Prepare the Steamer:**

   - Set up a steaming apparatus. This could be a bamboo steamer, an electric steamer, or a stovetop steamer.

2. **Season the Salmon:**

- Season the salmon fillets with salt and pepper. Place lemon slices and fresh herbs on top of the fillets for added flavor.

3. **Steam:**

   - Bring the water in the steamer to a gentle simmer. Place the salmon fillets in the steamer basket, ensuring they are not overcrowded.

4. **Cover and Steam:**

   - Cover the steamer with a lid. Steam the salmon for approximately 8-10 minutes, depending on the thickness of the fillets. The salmon is done when it easily flakes with a fork.

5. **Serve:**

- Carefully remove the salmon from the steamer. Serve the steamed fillets with additional lemon wedges and fresh herbs.

Tips:

- Experiment with different citrus slices or add a splash of white wine to the steaming liquid for additional flavor.

- Ensure that the steamer is well-sealed to prevent steam from escaping, maintaining an even cooking temperature.

Benefits of Steaming Salmon:

1. **Retains Nutrients:**

- Steaming preserves the nutritional integrity of

salmon by minimizing nutrient loss during cooking.

2. **Preserves Moisture:**

   - The gentle cooking process of steaming helps the salmon retain its natural moisture, resulting in a tender and succulent texture.

3. **Delicate Flavor:**

   - Steaming allows the subtle flavors of the salmon to shine through without overpowering them with additional seasonings or cooking methods.

4. **Healthy Cooking:**

- This cooking technique
  requires minimal added
  fats, making it a healthy
  and low-calorie option
  for salmon preparation.

Incorporating the steaming method into your culinary repertoire, you unlock a delicious and health-conscious way to enjoy the goodness of salmon. Whether for a light weeknight dinner or as part of a more elaborate meal, steamed salmon offers a delicate and nutritious dining experience.

CHAPTER 4

Simple Salmon Recipes for Beginners

Baking salmon is a straightforward yet delicious method that allows the natural flavors of the fish to shine. This Lemon Garlic Baked Salmon recipe is not only easy for beginners but also packs a punch of flavor. Let's dive into the details:

4.1 Lemon Garlic Baked Salmon

Ingredients:

- 4 salmon fillets

- 2 tablespoons olive oil

- 4 cloves garlic, minced

- 1 lemon, zest and juice

- 1 teaspoon dried oregano

- Salt and pepper, to taste

- Fresh parsley, chopped (for garnish)

Instructions:

1. **Preheat the Oven:**

   - Preheat your oven to 375°F (190°C).

2. **Prepare the Salmon:**

   - Pat the salmon fillets dry with paper towels. Place them on a baking sheet lined with parchment paper or aluminum foil.

3. **Make the Lemon Garlic Mixture:**

- In a small bowl, combine the olive oil, minced garlic, lemon zest, lemon juice, dried oregano, salt, and pepper. Mix well to create a flavorful marinade.

4. **Coat the Salmon:**

   - Brush the lemon garlic mixture evenly over each salmon fillet, ensuring they are well-coated on all sides.

5. **Bake in the Oven:**

   - Place the baking sheet in the preheated oven and bake for 12-15 minutes, or until the salmon easily flakes with a fork. Cooking times may vary based on the thickness of the fillets.

6. **Garnish and Serve:**

   - Once baked, remove the salmon from the oven. Garnish with chopped fresh parsley for a burst of color and freshness.

7. **Serve with Sides:**

   - Pair the Lemon Garlic Baked Salmon with your favorite sides such as steamed vegetables, roasted potatoes, or a simple green salad.

Tips:

- Adjust the level of garlic and lemon to suit your taste preferences.

- Consider marinating the salmon in the lemon garlic mixture for 30 minutes before baking for an extra flavor boost.

This Lemon Garlic Baked Salmon recipe not only introduces beginners to the ease of baking salmon but also provides a delightful combination of zesty and savory flavors. It's a perfect starting point for those looking to create a delicious and impressive salmon dish without the complexity of advanced culinary techniques.

4.2 Teriyaki Grilled Salmon

Grilling salmon with a sweet and savory teriyaki glaze adds an Asian-inspired flair to your culinary repertoire. This Teriyaki Grilled Salmon recipe is both simple for beginners and bursting with delicious flavors. Let's get started:

Ingredients:

- 4 salmon fillets

- 1/2 cup soy sauce

- 1/4 cup mirin (sweet rice wine)

- 2 tablespoons honey

- 1 tablespoon rice vinegar

- 2 cloves garlic, minced

- 1 teaspoon ginger, grated

- Sesame seeds (for garnish)

- Green onions, chopped (for garnish)

Instructions:

1. **Prepare the Teriyaki Marinade:**

- In a bowl, whisk together the soy sauce, mirin, honey, rice vinegar, minced garlic, and grated ginger to create the teriyaki marinade.

2. **Marinate the Salmon:**

   - Place the salmon fillets in a shallow dish or a resealable plastic bag. Pour half of the teriyaki marinade over the salmon, ensuring each fillet is well-coated. Reserve the remaining marinade for later.

3. **Marinate Time:**

   - Allow the salmon to marinate for at least 30 minutes, allowing the flavors to infuse into the fish. You can refrigerate it during this time.

4. **Preheat the Grill:**

    - Preheat your grill to medium-high heat. Make sure the grates are clean and well-oiled.

5. **Grilling:**

    - Remove the salmon from the marinade and discard the used marinade. Place the salmon fillets on the preheated grill. Grill for 4-5 minutes on each side, or until the salmon is opaque and easily flakes with a fork.

6. **Brush with Teriyaki Glaze:**

    - In the last few minutes of grilling, brush the

reserved teriyaki
marinade over the
salmon, creating a glossy
glaze.

7. **Garnish and Serve:**

   - Transfer the grilled
     salmon to a serving
     platter. Garnish with
     sesame seeds and
     chopped green onions for
     added flavor and visual
     appeal.

8. **Serve with Sides:**

   - Pair the Teriyaki Grilled
     Salmon with steamed
     rice, stir-fried vegetables,
     or a side of edamame for
     a complete and satisfying
     meal.

Tips:

- Adjust the sweetness or saltiness of the teriyaki marinade to your liking by tweaking the honey or soy sauce quantities.

- Consider adding a dash of sesame oil to the marinade for an extra layer of nutty flavor.

This Teriyaki Grilled Salmon recipe introduces beginners to the exciting world of grilled flavors with a delightful Asian twist. It's a perfect blend of simplicity and sophistication, making it an ideal dish for those looking to elevate their salmon-cooking skills.

4.3 Pan-Seared Lemon Butter Salmon

Pan-searing salmon with a luscious lemon butter sauce creates a dish that is both elegant and easy to prepare. This Pan-Seared Lemon Butter Salmon recipe is perfect for beginners, offering a burst of citrusy and rich flavors. Let's dive into the details:

Ingredients:

- 4 salmon fillets

- Salt and pepper, to taste

- 2 tablespoons olive oil

- 4 tablespoons unsalted butter

- 3 cloves garlic, minced

- Juice of 1 lemon

- 1 tablespoon fresh parsley, chopped (for garnish)

- Lemon wedges (for serving)

Instructions:

1. **Prepare the Salmon:**

   - Pat the salmon fillets dry with paper towels. Season both sides with salt and pepper.

2. **Heat the Pan:**

   - Heat a skillet or frying pan over medium-high heat. Add olive oil and let it heat until shimmering.

3. **Pan-Searing:**

   - Place the salmon fillets in the hot pan, skin-side down. Sear for 3-4

minutes until the skin
becomes crispy and
golden.

4. **Flip and Cook:**

   - Carefully flip the fillets
     using a spatula. Cook for
     an additional 3-4
     minutes, or until the
     salmon is opaque and
     flakes easily.

5. **Create Lemon Butter Sauce:**

   - Reduce the heat to
     medium-low. Add the
     butter and minced garlic
     to the pan. Allow the
     butter to melt and the
     garlic to sauté until
     fragrant.

6. **Lemon Infusion:**

- Squeeze the juice of one lemon into the pan, swirling it with the butter and garlic to create a rich lemon butter sauce.

7. **Baste the Salmon:**

   - Spoon the lemon butter sauce over the salmon fillets, ensuring they are coated evenly. Continue cooking for an additional 1-2 minutes.

8. **Garnish and Serve:**

   - Transfer the pan-seared salmon to a serving platter. Garnish with chopped fresh parsley and serve with lemon wedges on the side.

9. **Serve with Sides:**

- Pair the Pan-Seared
  Lemon Butter Salmon
  with sides like roasted
  vegetables, couscous, or
  a crisp green salad for a
  balanced meal.

Tips:

- For an extra burst of citrus, add
  lemon zest to the salmon before
  seasoning.

- Experiment with different herbs
  in the lemon butter sauce, such
  as thyme or dill.

This Pan-Seared Lemon Butter
Salmon recipe is a delightful
introduction to the art of pan-searing
and creating a flavorful sauce. With
its bright and buttery notes, this dish
elevates the classic pan-seared
salmon, making it a perfect choice for

those seeking a simple yet sophisticated culinary experience.

4.4 Easy Salmon Poke Bowl

Creating a Salmon Poke Bowl brings together the freshness of raw salmon with vibrant, wholesome ingredients. This recipe is not only easy for beginners but also customizable to suit individual tastes. Let's dive into crafting an Easy Salmon Poke Bowl

Ingredients:

- 2 cups sushi rice, cooked and seasoned with rice vinegar

- 1 pound fresh salmon, sushi-grade, diced

- 1 avocado, sliced

- 1 cucumber, julienned

- 1 cup edamame, steamed

- 1/4 cup soy sauce

- 1 tablespoon sesame oil

- 1 tablespoon honey

- 1 teaspoon grated ginger

- 1 teaspoon sesame seeds (optional)

- Nori strips (seaweed), for garnish

- Green onions, chopped, for garnish

Instructions:

1. **Prepare Sushi Rice:**

    - Cook the sushi rice according to package instructions. Once cooked, season with rice vinegar and let it cool to room temperature.

2. **Prepare Salmon:**

   - Ensure the salmon is fresh and sushi-grade. Dice the salmon into bite-sized cubes.

3. **Prepare Sauce:**

   - In a small bowl, whisk together soy sauce, sesame oil, honey, and grated ginger to create the sauce.

4. **Assemble the Poke Bowl:**

   - In serving bowls, arrange a portion of sushi rice as the base.

5. **Add Toppings:**

- Top the rice with diced salmon, sliced avocado, julienned cucumber, and steamed edamame.

6. **Drizzle with Sauce:**

   - Drizzle the prepared sauce over the ingredients in the bowl.

7. **Garnish:**

   - Garnish the bowl with sesame seeds (if using), nori strips, and chopped green onions.

8. **Mix and Enjoy:**

   - Gently mix the ingredients in the bowl to coat them with the sauce. Enjoy your easy Salmon Poke Bowl!

Tips:

- Customize your poke bowl with additional toppings like shredded carrots, radishes, or mango for a burst of sweetness.

- Experiment with different sauces, such as a spicy mayo or a ponzu-based dressing.

This Easy Salmon Poke Bowl is a vibrant and refreshing way to enjoy salmon. With its combination of fresh ingredients and a savory-sweet sauce, it's a delightful meal that requires minimal cooking and is perfect for those new to handling raw fish. The beauty of poke bowls lies in their versatility, allowing you to tailor them to your taste preferences.

4.5 Honey Mustard Glazed Salmon

A Honey Mustard Glazed Salmon recipe adds a delightful combination of sweet and tangy flavors to this versatile fish. This recipe is easy for beginners, offering a delicious twist to the classic salmon preparation. Let's explore how to make a Honey Mustard Glazed Salmon:

Ingredients:

- 4 salmon fillets
- Salt and pepper, to taste
- 2 tablespoons Dijon mustard
- 2 tablespoons honey
- 1 tablespoon whole-grain mustard
- 1 tablespoon olive oil

- 1 clove garlic, minced

- 1 teaspoon fresh lemon juice

- Lemon wedges (for serving)

- Fresh parsley, chopped (for garnish)

Instructions:

1. **Preheat the Oven:**

    - Preheat your oven to 375°F (190°C).

2. **Prepare the Salmon:**

    - Pat the salmon fillets dry with paper towels. Season both sides with salt and pepper.

3. **Create the Glaze:**

    - In a small bowl, whisk together Dijon mustard, honey, whole-grain

mustard, olive oil,
minced garlic, and fresh
lemon juice. This creates
the honey mustard glaze.

4. **Coat the Salmon:**

   - Place the salmon fillets
     on a baking sheet lined
     with parchment paper or
     aluminum foil. Brush the
     honey mustard glaze
     evenly over each fillet,
     ensuring they are well-
     coated.

5. **Bake in the Oven:**

   - Bake the salmon in the
     preheated oven for 12-15
     minutes, or until the
     salmon is opaque and
     flakes easily with a fork.

6. **Broil for Crispiness (Optional):**

   - If you desire a slightly caramelized and crispy top, you can broil the salmon for an additional 1-2 minutes, watching closely to prevent burning.

7. **Serve:**

   - Remove the Honey Mustard Glazed Salmon from the oven. Serve the fillets with lemon wedges on the side.

8. **Garnish:**

   - Garnish the salmon with chopped fresh parsley for a burst of color and freshness.

9. **Serve with Sides:**

- Pair the glazed salmon with your favorite sides such as roasted vegetables, quinoa, or a simple green salad.

Tips:

- Adjust the honey and mustard ratios to your taste preferences, creating a balance of sweetness and tanginess.

- For an extra layer of flavor, add a pinch of smoked paprika or dried herbs to the glaze.

This Honey Mustard Glazed Salmon recipe introduces beginners to the magic of a flavorful glaze that transforms a simple salmon dish into a culinary delight. With its sweet and savory notes, this recipe is a perfect addition to your repertoire of easy and impressive salmon preparations.

CHAPTER 5

Sides and Accompaniments

Enhancing the dining experience with well-chosen side dishes and salads can complement the flavors of salmon. Here's a guide to the best side dishes and salad pairings for salmon:

5.1 Best Side Dishes for Salmon

1. **Roasted Vegetables:**

   - Create a medley of colorful roasted vegetables such as asparagus, cherry tomatoes, and bell peppers. The caramelization from roasting adds a depth of flavor.

2. **Quinoa Pilaf:**

   - Prepare a quinoa pilaf with herbs, diced vegetables, and a squeeze of lemon. Quinoa is a nutrient-rich alternative to rice or couscous.

3. **Garlic Mashed Potatoes:**

   - Creamy garlic mashed potatoes complement the richness of salmon. Add roasted garlic for an extra layer of flavor.

4. **Grilled Asparagus:**

   - Lightly seasoned and grilled asparagus spears

provide a crisp and vibrant side that pairs well with the fish.

5. **Lemon Herb Rice:**

   - Infuse white or brown rice with fresh herbs like parsley and dill, and a squeeze of lemon juice for a citrusy lift.

6. **Sweet Potato Wedges:**

   - Roast sweet potato wedges with a sprinkle of cinnamon or paprika for a sweet and savory side dish.

7. **Sautéed Spinach:**

   - Quickly sautéed spinach with garlic and a dash of lemon is a light and nutritious option that

complements the
salmon's richness.

8. **Cucumber Avocado Salad:**

   - Toss together diced
     cucumber and creamy
     avocado with a simple
     vinaigrette for a
     refreshing side.

9. **Wild Rice Salad:**

   - Combine cooked wild
     rice with dried fruits,
     nuts, and a light
     vinaigrette for a hearty
     and flavorful salad.

10. **Steamed Broccoli:**

   - Steam broccoli until
     tender-crisp and drizzle
     with a lemon-infused
     olive oil for a simple and
     nutritious side.

5.2 Salad Pairings

1. **Citrus Kale Salad:**

   - Massage kale leaves with olive oil, then toss with segments of orange or grapefruit, sliced almonds, and a citrus vinaigrette.

2. **Caprese Salad:**

   - Pair salmon with a classic Caprese salad featuring fresh tomatoes, mozzarella, basil, and a balsamic glaze.

3. **Mango Avocado Salad:**

   - Combine diced mango, avocado, red onion, and cilantro for a vibrant and tropical salad that complements the salmon's flavors.

4. **Greek Salad:**

   - Create a Greek salad with cucumber, cherry tomatoes, Kalamata olives, feta cheese, and a lemon-oregano dressing.

5. **Arugula and Parmesan Salad:**

   - Toss peppery arugula with shaved Parmesan, pine nuts, and a lemony vinaigrette for a simple yet sophisticated side.

6. **Orzo Salad:**

   - Mix cooked orzo with cherry tomatoes, feta cheese, and a light Mediterranean dressing

for a versatile and
flavorful side dish.

7. **Asian Sesame Cucumber
Salad:**

- Combine thinly sliced
  cucumbers with sesame
  seeds and a soy-ginger
  dressing for a refreshing
  and crunchy salad.

8. **Watermelon Feta Salad:**

- Pair grilled salmon with
  a refreshing salad
  featuring watermelon,
  feta cheese, mint, and a
  balsamic glaze.

9. **Caesar Salad:**

- A classic Caesar salad
  with crisp romaine
  lettuce, Parmesan cheese,
  croutons, and Caesar

dressing is a timeless companion to salmon.

10. **Spinach and Strawberry Salad:**

- Toss fresh spinach with sliced strawberries, goat cheese, and candied nuts, drizzled with a balsamic vinaigrette for a sweet and savory combination.

These side dishes and salad pairings provide a range of textures and flavors that complement the richness of salmon. Whether you prefer roasted vegetables, grain salads, or refreshing greens, these accompaniments enhance the overall dining experience and add variety to your salmon-centric meals.

5.3 Rice and Grain Options

Pairing salmon with the right rice or grain can elevate the meal, providing a satisfying and balanced experience. Here are some versatile rice and grain options to complement your salmon dishes:

1. **Basmati Rice:**

   - Known for its fragrant aroma and fluffy texture, basmati rice is a classic choice that pairs well with a variety of salmon preparations.

2. **Jasmine Rice:**

   - Jasmine rice has a slightly sticky texture and a subtle floral aroma, making it an excellent companion to salmon dishes.

3. **Brown Rice:**

- For a nuttier flavor and added nutritional benefits, consider serving salmon with brown rice. It's a wholesome choice that complements the richness of the fish.

4. **Quinoa:**

- Quinoa is a protein-rich grain that works well with salmon. Its light and fluffy texture make it a versatile base for various salmon toppings and sauces.

5. **Wild Rice:**

- A blend of different rice varieties, wild rice has a chewy texture and a robust, nutty flavor that adds depth to salmon dishes.

6. **Couscous:**

    - Quick-cooking couscous is a convenient option that pairs well with salmon. It's light and can absorb the flavors of sauces and seasonings.

7. **Farro:**

    - Farro is a hearty ancient grain with a chewy texture. Its nutty flavor adds a rustic element to salmon dishes.

8. **Barley:**

- Barley has a chewy texture and a slightly nutty taste, making it a wholesome choice to accompany salmon.

9. **Bulgur:**

- Bulgur is a quick-cooking grain that adds a chewy texture to the plate. It's a great alternative for those seeking a nutritious side.

10. **Orzo:**

- Orzo, a rice-shaped pasta, is a versatile option that works well in salads or as a side dish with salmon.

11. **Forbidden Rice (Black Rice):**

- Forbidden rice has a striking deep purple color and a nutty flavor. It's a visually appealing and nutritious choice to serve with salmon.

12. **Millet:**

- Millet is a gluten-free grain with a mild flavor and a fluffy texture. It's a great option for those looking to diversify their grain choices.

Tips for Cooking Rice and Grains:

- **Rinse Before Cooking:**

  - Rinse rice or grains under cold water before cooking to remove excess starch, ensuring a fluffier result.

- **Use Broth or Stock:**

  - Cook rice or grains in vegetable or chicken broth to infuse them with additional flavor.

- **Add Fresh Herbs or Citrus:**

  - Enhance the aroma and flavor of rice or grains by adding fresh herbs, such as parsley or dill, or a squeeze of citrus.

- **Experiment with Spices:**

  - Season rice or grains with spices like cumin, coriander, or turmeric to add depth to the dish.

Choosing the right rice or grain to accompany your salmon, you can create a well-balanced and satisfying meal. Experiment with different

options to find your favorite pairings
and enjoy the diverse textures and
flavors that each grain brings to the
table.

CHAPTER 6

Tips for Success

Achieving the perfect salmon dish involves mastering various aspects of cooking, seasoning, and handling leftovers. Here are some tips to ensure success in preparing and enjoying your salmon:

6.1 Cooking Times and Temperatures

1. **Know the Thickness:**

   - Adjust cooking times based on the thickness of your salmon fillets. Thicker cuts may require

a few extra minutes in
the oven or on the grill.

2. **Use a Meat Thermometer:**

    - Invest in a meat
      thermometer to ensure
      precise cooking. Salmon
      is cooked when its
      internal temperature
      reaches 145°F (63°C).

3. **Avoid Overcooking:**

    - Overcooked salmon can
      become dry. Aim for a
      slightly translucent
      center for a moist and
      tender result.

4. **Grilling Tips:**

    - Preheat the grill before
      cooking. Oil the grates to
      prevent sticking, and grill

skin-side down first for a crispy finish.

5. **Baking Perfection:**

   - When baking salmon, use parchment paper or aluminum foil to prevent sticking and make cleanup easier.

6.2 Seasoning and Flavoring Tips

1. **Experiment with Marinades:**

   - Marinate salmon for at least 30 minutes before cooking to infuse it with flavor. Common marinade ingredients include soy sauce, citrus juices, herbs, and olive oil.

2. **Balanced Seasoning:**

- Season salmon with a balance of salt and pepper. Consider adding complementary flavors such as garlic, lemon, dill, or paprika.

3. **Citrus Brightens Flavors:**

- Citrus, especially lemon, enhances the natural flavors of salmon. Squeeze fresh lemon juice over the fish before or after cooking.

4. **Herbs for Freshness:**

- Fresh herbs like dill, parsley, and cilantro add a burst of freshness. Sprinkle them over the

salmon just before
serving.

5. **Try Dry Rubs:**

  - Dry rubs, made with a
    mix of spices and herbs,
    can create a flavorful
    crust when applied to
    salmon before cooking.

6.3 Handling Leftover Salmon

1. **Refrigerate Promptly:**

  - Store leftover salmon in
    the refrigerator within
    two hours of cooking.
    Place it in an airtight
    container to maintain
    freshness.

2. **Use Within 3 Days:**

- Consume leftover salmon within three days. Consider incorporating it into salads, wraps, or pasta dishes for a quick and tasty meal.

3. **Reheat Gently:**

   - When reheating, do so gently to prevent drying out the salmon. Use methods like low-temperature baking, steaming, or microwaving with a damp paper towel.

4. **Flavor Boost:**

   - Add a splash of lemon juice or a drizzle of olive oil when reheating to revive flavors.

5. **Creative Leftover Ideas:**

- Transform leftover salmon into salmon cakes, a filling for sandwiches, or a topping for salads to avoid monotony.

Paying attention to cooking times, experimenting with seasonings, and effectively handling leftovers, you can ensure that your salmon dishes are consistently delicious and enjoyable. Whether you're a beginner or a seasoned cook, these tips will help you master the art of preparing and savoring this versatile and nutritious fish.

CHAPTER 7
Exploring Advanced Salmon Recipes

Taking your salmon culinary skills to the next level involves exploring advanced cooking techniques and flavors. Here are three sophisticated salmon recipes to add to your repertoire:

7.1 Salmon en Papillote

Ingredients:

- 4 salmon fillets

- Salt and pepper, to taste

- 2 tablespoons olive oil

- 1 lemon, thinly sliced

- 1 fennel bulb, thinly sliced

- 4 sprigs fresh dill

- 1/4 cup white wine

Instructions:

1. **Preheat the Oven:**

   - Preheat your oven to 400°F (200°C).

2. **Prepare Parchment Packets:**

   - Cut four large squares of parchment paper. Place a salmon fillet on each square and season with salt and pepper.

3. **Layer Ingredients:**

- Drizzle olive oil over each fillet. Arrange lemon slices, fennel slices, and fresh dill on top. Pour a tablespoon of white wine over each fillet.

4. **Seal Packets:**

   - Fold the parchment paper over the salmon and ingredients, creating a sealed packet. Crimp the edges to ensure it's well-sealed.

5. **Bake:**

   - Place the sealed packets on a baking sheet and bake in the preheated oven for 12-15 minutes, or until the salmon is cooked through.

6. **Serve:**

   - Carefully open the
     packets at the table,
     allowing the aromatic
     steam to escape. Serve
     the salmon directly from
     the parchment for an
     elegant presentation.

7.2 Cedar Plank Salmon

Ingredients:

- 4 salmon fillets

- Salt and pepper, to taste

- 1 cedar plank, soaked in water
  for at least 1 hour

- 2 tablespoons Dijon mustard

- 2 tablespoons maple syrup

- 1 tablespoon soy sauce

- 1 teaspoon grated ginger

Instructions:

1. **Prepare the Cedar Plank:**

   - Soak the cedar plank in water for at least 1 hour to prevent it from burning during grilling.

2. **Season Salmon:**

   - Season the salmon fillets with salt and pepper on both sides.

3. **Mix the Glaze:**

   - In a small bowl, whisk together Dijon mustard, maple syrup, soy sauce, and grated ginger to create the glaze.

4. **Brush with Glaze:**

- Brush the cedar plank
  with a bit of the glaze.
  Place the salmon fillets
  on the cedar plank and
  brush the tops with the
  remaining glaze.

5. **Grill:**

  - Preheat the grill to
    medium-high heat. Place
    the cedar plank with
    salmon on the grill and
    close the lid. Grill for 12-
    15 minutes or until the
    salmon is cooked
    through.

6. **Serve:**

  - Carefully remove the
    cedar plank from the grill
    and serve the salmon
    directly from the plank

for a smoky and flavorful experience.

7.3 Salmon Ceviche

Ingredients:

- 1 pound sushi-grade salmon, diced

- 1/2 red onion, finely diced

- 1 cucumber, diced

- 1 avocado, diced

- 1 jalapeño, seeded and finely chopped

- 1/4 cup fresh cilantro, chopped

- Juice of 4 limes

- Salt and pepper, to taste

- Tortilla chips (for serving)

Instructions:

1. **Prepare Salmon:**

   - In a bowl, combine diced salmon with red onion, cucumber, avocado, jalapeño, and cilantro.

2. **Add Lime Juice:**

   - Squeeze the juice of 4 limes over the ingredients. Mix well to ensure the salmon is evenly coated with lime juice.

3. **Season:**

   - Season the ceviche with salt and pepper to taste. Adjust the seasoning as needed.

4. **Chill:**

- Cover the bowl with plastic wrap and refrigerate for at least 30 minutes to allow the flavors to meld and the salmon to "cook" in the lime juice.

5. **Serve:**

- Serve the salmon ceviche in individual bowls with tortilla chips on the side for scooping. Enjoy this refreshing and zesty dish as an appetizer or light meal.

These advanced salmon recipes showcase different cooking methods and flavor profiles. From the delicate and aromatic Salmon en Papillote to the smoky Cedar Plank Salmon and the vibrant and citrusy Salmon

Ceviche, these recipes provide a
glimpse into the diverse and
sophisticated world of salmon cuisine.